GLORIOUSTINA ESSIA

Nature's Apothecary: Crafting Herbal Remedies at Home"

A Comprehensive Guide to Creating Natural Tinctures, Infusions, Oils, and More for Health and Healing

Contents

INTRODUCTION

Welcome to "Nature's Apothecary," the third enlightening volume in the **"Green Healing: The Natural Medicine Bible"** series, where the ancient art of herbal remedy preparation is brought into your home. This book is a treasure trove for those seeking to harness the healing powers of plants, offering a hands-on approach to creating your natural tinctures, infusions, oils, and more.

In an era where the quest for natural health solutions is ever-growing, "Nature's Apothecary" is a beacon of knowledge and empowerment. It demystifies the process of herbal remedy preparation, guiding you through the intricate steps of crafting potent and effective natural medicines. From the soothing calm of chamomile tea to the healing embrace of lavender-infused oil, this book unveils the secrets to unlocking the full potential of herbs for health and wellness.

As part of the "Green Healing" series, this guide deepens your understanding of herbal properties and fosters a profound connection with the natural world. You will learn to blend tradition with modernity as each page weaves the age-old wisdom of herbal remedies with contemporary techniques and insights.

Embark on this journey of discovery and transformation, where each herb you nurture, and each remedy you craft brings you closer to the heart of nature's apothecary. "Nature's Apothecary: Crafting Herbal Remedies at Home" is more than a guide; it's your companion on the path to natural wellness, echoing the ethos of a life attuned to nature's rhythms and remedies.

Join us in unfolding the pages of herbal mastery, where every recipe and instruction opens doors to a healthier, more natural way of living. Embrace the art of creating your herbal remedies and let "Nature's Apothecary" guide the enriching world of natural healing.

CHAPTER 1: ESSENTIALS OF HERB PREPARATION

The preparation of herbs is crucial in unlocking their medicinal and culinary potential. This chapter covers the foundational techniques for preparing herbs, ensuring you can effectively utilize their benefits.

Understanding Different Forms of Herbal Preparations

Herbal remedies can be prepared in various forms, each serving a specific purpose and offering different benefits.

- **Teas and Infusions:** Ideal for delicate parts of the plant, like leaves, flowers, and fine stems. For example, chamomile tea infuses the flowers in hot water, making a soothing drink that aids relaxation.
- **Decoctions:** Used for tougher plant materials like roots, bark, and seeds. Decoctions involve simmering the plant material in water for a longer period. For instance, a ginger root decoction can be used for its anti-inflammatory properties.
- **Tinctures:** These are concentrated herbal extracts made by soaking herbs in alcohol. Tinctures have a long shelf life and allow for easy dosage control. Echinacea tincture, for example, is commonly used to boost the immune system.
- **Salves and Ointments:** These are topical preparations made by infusing

herbs in oils and mixing them with beeswax. Calendula salve is popular for its skin-healing properties.

Proper Techniques for Drying Herbs

Drying is fundamental for preserving herbs, concentrating their flavors and active compounds.

- **Air Drying:** Suitable for most herbs, this method involves hanging bunches upside down in a warm, dry, and well-ventilated area. Herbs like oregano, thyme, and sage are ideal for air drying.
- **Oven Drying:** This faster method is useful for herbs that might mold if air-dried. Spread the herbs on a baking sheet and dry them in an oven at the lowest setting, checking frequently to prevent burning.
- **Dehydrator Drying:** A dehydrator provides a controlled environment for drying herbs, ideal for those with high moisture content like basil or mint.

Creating Herbal Infusions and Decoctions

Infusions and decoctions extract the medicinal properties of herbs using water.

- **Preparing Infusions:** Place dried or fresh herbs in a teapot or jar, pour boiling water over them, and let them steep. The steeping time varies depending on the herb.
- **Making Decoctions:** Place the plant material in a pot, cover it with cold water, slowly bring it to a boil, and then simmer for an extended period, usually between 20 minutes and an hour. This method effectively extracts the deeper essence from tougher materials like roots and bark.

Tincture Preparation

Tinctures offer a convenient and long-lasting way to consume herbs.

- **Basic Process:** Chop or grind the dried herb, place it in a jar, and cover it with a solvent, typically alcohol. The jar is sealed and left to sit for several weeks, shaking it periodically.
- **Straining and Storage:** After the steeping period, strain the liquid, squeezing as much as possible from the herb material. Store the tincture in amber or blue glass droppers for easy use and protection from light.

Making Herbal Oils, Salves, and Balms

Topical herbal preparations are excellent for skin conditions, wounds, and muscle aches.

- **Herbal Oils:** Infuse herbs in a carrier oil, like olive or almond oil, either by heating them together gently or letting them sit in a warm, sunny spot for several weeks.
- **Salves and Balms:** Once the infusion is ready, strain the oil and gently heat it with beeswax until the wax melts. Pour the mixture into containers and let it cool to solidify.

Quality Control in Herb Preparation

Ensuring the quality of your herbal preparations is crucial for their effectiveness.

- **Source High-Quality Herbs:** Whether growing your own or purchasing, ensure the herbs are high-quality, organically grown, and free from pesticides and contaminants.
- **Attention to Detail:** Be meticulous in your measurements, especially when making tinctures or oils, to ensure consistency and potency.

- **Storage and Shelf Life:** Store your preparations in a cool, dark place. Most tinctures last for several years, while dried herbs, oils, and salves generally have a shelf life of about a year.

Mastering the essentials of herb preparation allows you to tap into the full potential of your herb garden. From soothing teas to healing salves, each preparation method offers a unique way to enjoy the benefits of herbs. With patience, practice, and attention to detail, you can create a range of effective and natural remedies right in your home.

CHAPTER 2: MAKING HERBAL INFUSIONS AND DECOCTIONS

Herbal infusions and decoctions are traditional methods of extracting the therapeutic properties of herbs. This chapter explores these techniques in detail, guiding how to prepare these healing drinks effectively.

Herbal Infusions

Infusions are typically made with the more delicate parts of the plant, such as leaves, flowers, and light stems. They involve steeping the plant material in hot water.

Preparing Herbal Infusions:

1. **Selecting Herbs:** Choose fresh or dried herbs based on your desired effect, such as peppermint for digestion or chamomile for relaxation.
2. **Proportion and Water Temperature:** A general guideline is to use one teaspoon of dried or one tablespoon of fresh herbs per cup of boiling water. The water temperature should be just off the boil to preserve the delicate compounds in the herbs.
3. **Steeping Time:** The steeping time can vary depending on the herb. Generally, it ranges from 5 to 15 minutes. Longer steeping times extract more nutrients but can release more tannins, making the infusion bitter.
4. **Straining and Serving:** Strain the herbs from the infusion and serve.

Honey, lemon, or other natural sweeteners can be added to taste. **Storage:** Freshly made infusions are best consumed immediately but can be refrigerated for up to 24 hours. After that, the potency and flavor may start to diminish.

Herbal Decoctions

Decoctions are used for the tougher parts of the plant, like roots, barks, seeds, and berries. They involve simmering the plant material in water over a longer period.

Preparing Herbal Decoctions:

1. **Choosing Herbs:** Select appropriate herbs, such as ginger root for digestion or valerian root for sleep.
2. **Preparing the Herbs:** Chop or grind the plant material to increase the surface area. This helps in extracting more active compounds.
3. **Water Quantity and Boiling:** A general ratio is one part herb to eight parts water. Bring the water to a boil, then add the herbs.
4. **Simmering:** Reduce the heat and let the mixture simmer. Depending on the herb, this can take about 20 minutes to an hour. The liquid should be reduced by about one-third.
5. **Straining and Storing:** Strain the decoction, and it's ready to drink. Like infusions, decoctions are best consumed fresh but can be stored in the refrigerator for up to 48 hours.

Tips for Maximizing Efficacy

- **Quality of Herbs:** Always use organic herbs to ensure the best results. The potency of the infusion or decoction greatly depends on the quality of the starting material.
- **Ratio Adjustments:** The ratio of herbs to water depends on the desired strength. Medicinal decoctions, for example, require a higher concentration of herbs.

- **Combining Herbs:** You can combine different herbs in one infusion or decoction to target specific health issues. For instance, combining lavender and chamomile can enhance relaxation effects.
- **Culinary Uses:** Herbal infusions and decoctions can also be used in cooking. For example, a rosemary infusion can add flavor to soups or stews.

Caution and Considerations

- **Medical Interactions:** Be aware of potential interactions between herbs and medications. Consult with a healthcare provider if you are on medication or have underlying health conditions.

CHAPTER 3: CRAFTING TINCTURES AND EXTRACTS

Tinctures and extracts are concentrated herbal preparations made by soaking herbs in a solvent, typically alcohol. They are valued for their long shelf life and ease of use. This chapter provides an extensive guide on how to craft these potent remedies.

Understanding Tinctures and Extracts

- **Tinctures** are alcohol-based extracts that efficiently pull out the active compounds from herbs. They are typically more diluted than pure extracts.
- **Extracts** are similar to tinctures but are often more concentrated and can use solvents other than alcohol, such as glycerin or vinegar.

Choosing the Right Herbs and Solvents

- **Selecting Herbs:** Virtually any herb can make a tincture, but some popular choices include echinacea for immune support, valerian root for sleep aid, and milk thistle for liver health.
- **Choosing Solvents:** The most common solvent is alcohol, such as vodka or brandy, due to its efficiency in extracting various plant constituents. For alcohol-free tinctures, glycerin or apple cider vinegar are good alternatives, though they may only extract some compounds as effectively

as alcohol.

Preparing and Making Tinctures

- **Proportions:** A common ratio for tinctures is 1:4 for dried herbs (one part herb to four parts solvent) or 1:2 for fresh herbs.
- **Maceration:** Finely chop or grind the herbs to increase the surface area. Please place them in a clean jar and pour the solvent over them, ensuring they are completely covered.
- **Steeping:** Seal the jar and store it in a cool, dark place for about 4 to 6 weeks. Shake the jar daily to help the extraction process.
- **Straining:** Strain the tincture through a fine mesh strainer or cheesecloth after steeping. Squeeze or press the herb matter to extract as much liquid as possible.
- **Bottling and Labeling:** Transfer the strained tincture into dark glass dropper bottles for storage. Label each bottle with the herb name, type of solvent used, and the date of preparation.

Preparing and Making Extracts

- **Concentration:** Extracts are often more concentrated than tinctures. The ratio can vary depending on the desired strength, but a common starting point is a 1:1 ratio.
- **Extended Maceration:** Some extracts may benefit from longer steeping times, up to several months, to fully concentrate the active compounds.
- **Reducing and Concentrating:** For a more concentrated extract, gently heat the strained liquid to reduce its volume. This should be done at a low temperature to preserve the integrity of the compounds.

Storing Tinctures and Extracts

- **Storage Conditions:** Store in a cool, dark place. Sunlight and heat can degrade the quality of the tincture or extract.
- **Shelf Life:** Alcohol-based tinctures can last several years. Glycerin-based tinctures and vinegar extracts have a shorter shelf life, typically around 1-2 years.

Using Tinctures and Extracts

- **Dosage:** The appropriate dosage can vary greatly depending on the herb, the strength of the tincture or extract, and the individual's needs. Start with a low dose, often a few drops, and increase as needed.
- **Administration:** Tinctures and extracts can be taken directly under the tongue for fast absorption or added to water, tea, or juice.
- **Culinary Uses:** Some tinctures, particularly those made with culinary herbs, can be used in cooking and baking as flavor enhancers.

Safety and Precautions

Alcohol Content: Be mindful of the alcohol content in tinctures, especially when using them for children, pregnant women, or individuals with alcohol sensitivities.

- **Herb Interactions:** Research potential interactions between the herb in your tincture and medications or conditions you may have.
- **Quality of Ingredients:** Use high-quality, organic herbs and solvents to ensure the purity and efficacy of your tinctures and extracts.
- **Testing and Adjusting:** Start with small doses to test for adverse reactions and adjust the dosage as needed.

Advanced Techniques

- **Combining Herbs:** You can create compound tinctures by combining multiple herbs that work synergistically for a specific therapeutic effect. For example, a tincture combining chamomile, lavender, and valerian can be effective for relaxation and sleep aid.
- **Percolation Method:** For more experienced herbalists, the percolation method is a quicker way to prepare tinctures, using a percolator to pass solvent through the herbs, which takes only a day or two.
- **Standardization:** Some herbalists aim for standardization in their tinctures to ensure consistent potency. This involves measuring the concentration of certain active ingredients and adjusting the preparation process accordingly. However, this requires advanced knowledge and equipment.

Creative Applications

- **Topical Use:** Some tinctures can be used topically, directly, or in creams and salves for conditions like skin irritations or muscle pain.
- **Herbal Sprays:** Tinctures can be diluted and used in spray form for throat sprays or easy topical applications.
- **Gifts and Custom Blends:** Homemade tinctures and extracts make thoughtful, personalized gifts. Creating custom blends for friends and family can be creative and rewarding.

In summary, crafting tinctures and extracts is a valuable skill for anyone interested in herbal medicine. It allows for the preservation and convenient use of medicinal herbs and offers flexibility in dosage and application. With practice, you can create a range of potent, natural remedies tailored to your specific health needs and preferences.

CHAPTER 4: CREATING SALVES, OILS AND BALMS

Creating salves, oils, and balms is a rewarding process that allows you to harness the healing properties of herbs in topical forms. These preparations address various skin issues, from dryness and irritation to cuts and bruises. This chapter will guide you through making herbal salves, oils, and balms.

Herbal Oils

Herbal oils are the foundation of many topical preparations and can be used directly on the skin or as a base for salves and balms.

- **Infusing Oils with Herbs:** Choose a carrier oil like olive, almond, or coconut. Place dried herbs in the oil and allow them to infuse. There are two main methods:
- **Cold Infusion:** Combine herbs and oil in a jar and let it sit in a sunny spot for 2-4 weeks, shaking daily.
- **Heat Infusion:** Gently heat the herb and oil mixture in a double boiler for 2-3 hours, ensuring the oil does not overheat.
- **Straining:** Once the infusion is complete, strain the oil through the cheesecloth to remove the herb particles. Store the infused oil in a cool, dark place.

Making Herbal Salves

Salves are thicker than oils and are excellent for treating targeted areas on the skin.

- **Ingredients:** To make a salve, you need infused herbal oil, beeswax, and, optionally, essential oils for added therapeutic benefits and fragrance.
- **Proportions and Process:** A general guideline is to use about 1 part beeswax to 4-8 parts infused oil, depending on how firm you want the salve. Gently heat the beeswax and herbal oil together until the beeswax melts. Pour the mixture into containers and let it cool.
- **Examples:** Calendula salve is popular for soothing skin irritations, and arnica salve is used for bruises and muscle aches.

Crafting Herbal Balms

Balms are similar to salves but often have a higher concentration of beeswax, making them firmer.

- **Texture and Ingredients:** For extra nourishment, Balms may include additional ingredients like shea butter or cocoa butter. This makes them ideal for lip balms or more intensive skin treatments.
- **Preparation:** The process for making balms is similar to salves. Melt the beeswax, carrier oil, and butter together, then pour the mixture into containers to set.
- **Examples:** Peppermint lip balm for chapped lips or a lavender and chamomile balm for soothing stress and aiding sleep.

Quality Control and Storage

- **Purity of Ingredients:** Use high-quality, preferably organic herbs and carrier oils. The quality of your ingredients directly affects the potency and effectiveness of the final product.

- **Storage:** Store salves and balms in a cool, dark place. Tins or small glass jars are ideal containers. Properly stored, they can last for up to a year.

Safety and Testing

- **Patch Testing:** Before using any new topical preparation, it's wise to do a patch test, especially if you have sensitive skin or are prone to allergies. Apply a small amount of the product to a discreet skin area and wait 24 hours to check for any adverse reactions.
- **Preservatives:** While most salves and balms do not require preservatives due to their low moisture content, be cautious if you include water-based ingredients. These can introduce bacteria and may require the use of natural preservatives.

Customization and Creativity

- **Tailoring to Needs:** You can customize salves and balms according to specific needs. For instance, add tea tree oil for its antiseptic properties or chamomile for its soothing effect.
- **Experimentation:** Don't hesitate to experiment with different herb and oil combinations. Each herb has unique properties, and part of the joy of making your products is discovering what works best for you.

Hence, making herbal salves, oils, and balms is a practical skill and a deeply satisfying way to connect with nature and care for your body. These herbal preparations offer a natural, chemical-free alternative to store-bought skin care products. They can be tailored to specific skin types and conditions, and their preparation allows for creativity and experimentation with different herbs and oils. With some basic knowledge and simple ingredients, you can create a range of personalized, effective, and natural skin care remedies.

CHAPTER 5: ADVANCED PREPARATION TECHNIQUES

Beyond the basic methods of preparing herbal remedies, advanced techniques can enhance your preparations' potency, specificity, and shelf-life. These methods often require specialized knowledge and equipment but can lead to more sophisticated and targeted herbal products.

Distillation for Essential Oils and Hydrosols

Distillation extracts essential oils and hydrosols (floral waters) from herbs.

- **Essential Oils:** These are highly concentrated plant extracts obtained by steam distilling the volatile compounds from herbs. For example, distilling lavender produces a potent essential oil for relaxation and stress relief.
- **Hydrosols:** Also known as floral waters, hydrosols are the water-based byproducts of the distillation process. They contain the water-soluble constituents of the herb and have milder effects. Rose water, a byproduct of distilling rose petals, is a popular hydrosol used in skincare.
- **Equipment and Process:** Distillation requires specific equipment, like a still. The plant material is heated with water, and the steam carries the volatile oils. The steam is then cooled, condensing the oil and water, and separated afterward.

Solvent Extraction for Concentrated Extracts

Solvent extraction creates highly concentrated extracts, often used in perfumery and aromatherapy.

- **Process:** This involves using solvents like ethanol or hexane to extract the aromatic compounds from herbs. The solvent is then removed, leaving behind the concentrated extract.
- **Applications:** Jasmine and vanilla are commonly extracted using this method, as they contain delicate aromatic compounds that are not easily extracted through distillation.

Maceration and Percolation Tinctures

Beyond the simple tincture preparation, there are more precise methods like maceration and percolation.

- **Maceration Tinctures:** This involves soaking the herb in a solvent over an extended period while regularly agitating the mixture. It's suitable for herbs that require longer extraction times.
- **Percolation Tinctures:** A more technical method, percolation involves passing a solvent through powdered herbs to create a tincture. This method is faster and often yields a more concentrated tincture.

Advanced Topical Preparations: Creams and Lotions

Creating herbal creams and lotions requires emulsification, which is the process of combining oil and water.

- **Emulsification** involves using natural emulsifiers like beeswax or lecithin to bind oil and water together. The process requires careful temperature control and mixing to achieve a stable emulsion.
- **Preservatives:** Since creams and lotions contain water, they are sus-

ceptible to bacterial growth. Natural preservatives like grapefruit seed extract or vitamin E can help extend shelf life.

- **Customization:** You can customize creams and lotions for specific skin types or conditions by selecting appropriate herbal infusions or essential oils. For example, a cream made with calendula-infused oil can be beneficial for soothing irritated skin.

Encapsulation and Pill-Making

Encapsulation involves preparing herbal remedies in a pill form, which can be more convenient for some users.

- **Powdering Herbs:** The first step is to powder the dried herbs finely. This can be done using a grinder or mill.
- **Capsule Machines:** Capsule machines can fill empty capsules with powdered herbs. This allows for precise dosing and convenient consumption.
- **Pill-Making:** Some herbs can be mixed with binding agents and formed into pills. This requires specific techniques to ensure the pills hold together and release their contents effectively when consumed.

Fermentation for Herbal Preparations

Fermentation can enhance the bioavailability and potency of certain herbal preparations.

- **Fermented Herbal Tonics:** Fermenting herbs in a medium like water or alcohol can create healthy tonics. Kombucha, for example, often incorporates herbs for additional health benefits.
- **Process:** The fermentation process allows beneficial bacteria and yeasts to break down the plant materials, often enhancing their nutritional profile and making them easier to digest.

Advanced Extraction Techniques: CO2 Extracts and Ultrasonication

- **CO2 Extracts:** Supercritical CO2 extraction is a method that uses carbon dioxide under high pressure to extract plant compounds. This method is highly efficient and can extract a wide range of compounds without heat, preserving the integrity of the plant's constituents.
- **Ultrasonication:** This method uses ultrasound waves to create rapid vibrations in the plant material, breaking down the cell walls and releasing active compounds. It's a fast, efficient way to extract herbal constituents.

These advanced preparation techniques allow for greater exploration and utilization of the medicinal properties of herbs. They can lead to more potent, refined, and specific herbal products catering to various needs and preferences. While some of these methods require specialized equipment and knowledge, they offer exciting possibilities for those looking to deepen their practice of herbal medicine.

CONCLUSION

As we conclude our journey through "Nature's Apothecary," part of the esteemed "Green Healing: The Natural Medicine Bible" series, we hope you carry with you not just the knowledge to craft herbal remedies but a deepened respect for the power and versatility of nature's bounty. This book has explored the heart of herbalism, an invitation to infuse your life with the wisdom and wellness that only nature can provide.

Throughout these pages, you've learned the art of transforming simple herbs into powerful healing agents, creating everything from soothing tinctures to revitalizing oils. This knowledge empowers you to take control of your health most naturally, blending ancient herbal practices with the needs of contemporary living.

But the journey doesn't end here. Each remedy you create and each herb you nurture is a step forward in your lifelong relationship with natural wellness. We encourage you to continue experimenting, learning, and growing in your herbal practice and journey towards holistic health.

Remember, "Nature's Apothecary" is more than just a book; it's a testament to the healing power of the natural world, a companion in your quest for a healthier, more balanced life. As you close this chapter, know that the world of herbal remedies is ever-evolving, just like the plants that inspire it.

May your path be evergreen, your health vibrant, and your spirit in harmony with the healing rhythms of nature. Embrace the wisdom of "Green Healing," and let the art of herbal remedy preparation enrich your life today and always.

SOURCES

https://www.healthline.com/health/herbal-medicine-101-harness-the-power-of-healing-herbs#trusted-retailers

https://www.healthline.com/health/herbal-medicine-101-harness-the-power-of-healing-herbs

https://nchfp.uga.edu/how/dry/herbs.html#:~:text=Drying%20is%20the%20easiest%20method,can%20lose%20flavor%20and%20color.

https://extension.psu.edu/lets-preserve-drying-herbs

https://www.bhg.com/gardening/vegetable/herbs/drying-herbs/

https://blog.mountainroseherbs.com/herbal-infusions-and-decoctions

https://www.homsted.com/blogs/homsted/how-to-make-an-herbal-tea-infusion-decoction/

https://www.fromnaturewithlove.com/library/infusion.asp

https://achs.edu/blog/2017/07/25/how-to-make-a-tincture-herbal-medicine/

https://earthsongseeds.co.uk/recipes/how-to-make-a-herbal-salve/

SOURCES

https://www.healthline.com/health/diy-herbal-salves

https://blog.mountainroseherbs.com/diy-herbal-salves

https://www.pharmatutor.org/pharmacognosy/quality-control-of-phytom
edicines.html

https://www.sciencedirect.com/science/article/pii/S2666831921000400

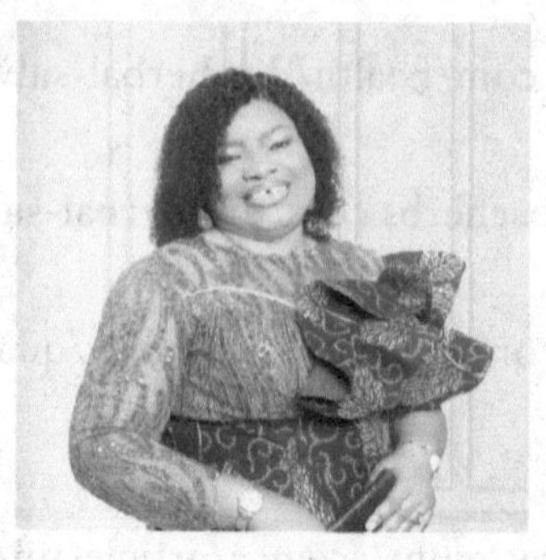

About the Author

Glorioustina Essia is a multifaceted professional whose expertise traverses the realms of technology, artificial intelligence, literature, and natural health. As a driving force in artificial intelligence, particularly in prompt engineering, she has established herself as a pioneer. Her proficiency extends to project management, network marketing, website development, and copywriting, showcasing a unique blend of technical understanding and creative flair.

A prolific author and publisher, Glorioustina's literary works span multiple genres, captivating a diverse audience with her narrative skill and inspiring a new generation of writers to unlock their creative potential. Her passion for storytelling matches her commitment to exploring and advocating for holistic health practices. Renowned in herbal medicine, she dedicates her life to studying and promoting natural health.

Glorioustina Essia's professional and personal journey is characterized by an unwavering dedication to her core strengths and a ceaseless pursuit of knowledge. Her zeal and expertise embody the limitless possibilities that arise from a commitment to innovation, quality, and a deep-seated passion for understanding the future of technology and the ancient wisdom of herbal medicine. Glorioustina is a testament to the power of interdisciplinary knowledge and its impact in a world where technology, literature, and natural health converge.

Also by Glorioustina Essia

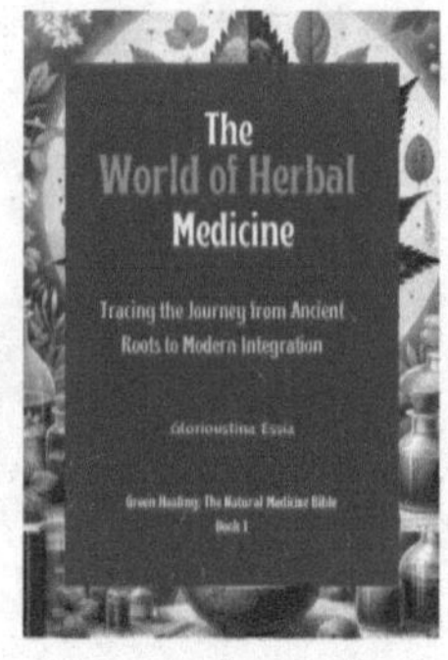

The World of Herbal Medicine
In an era where the rush of modern medicine often overshadows the pursuit of holistic health, the timeless wisdom of herbal remedies remains largely untapped. Do you find yourself seeking a more natural approach to health and wellness yet still determining where to begin or how to integrate these practices with modern healthcare?

Embark on a transformative journey with Book 1 of "Green Healing: The Natural Medicine Bible": "The World of Herbal Medicine." This enlightening volume takes you through the ancient pathways to the modern integration of herbal healing. Discover herbal medicine's rich history and evolution across different cultures, including the profound insights of Traditional Chinese Medicine, Ayurveda, and indigenous practices. Unravel how herbalism has evolved through historical epochs and how it beautifully intersects with modern medical practices today.

Embrace the journey to holistic health – add this captivating volume to your collection and begin exploring the world of herbal medicine today!

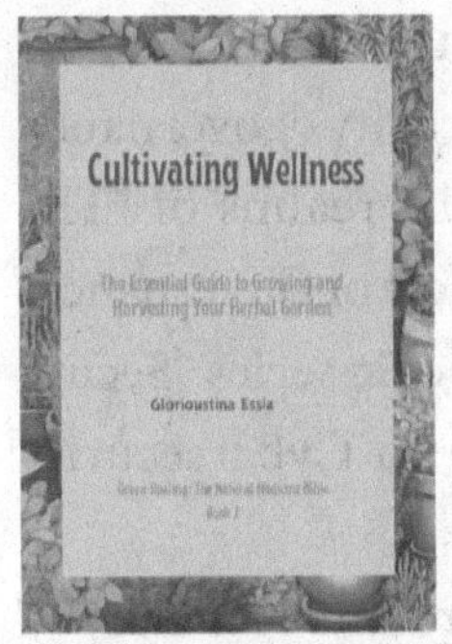

Cultivating Wellness

This guide is your gateway to mastering the art of herb gardening, offering practical advice for cultivating various medicinal and culinary herbs. From sustainable techniques to harvesting and preservation methods, each chapter brims with expert knowledge tailored to beginners and experienced gardeners. Learn to navigate common challenges in herb gardening and create specialized gardens for your health and culinary needs. Beyond gardening tips, this book inspires a deeper connection with nature and a commitment to a holistic lifestyle. Embrace the journey of nurturing not just a garden but a healthier, more harmonious way of life with "Cultivating Wellness."

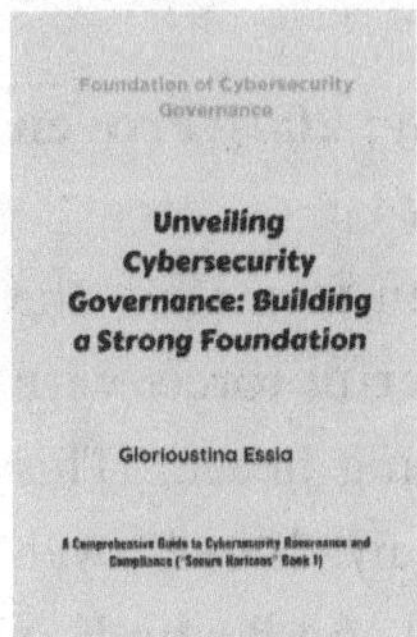

Unveiling Cybersecurity Governance

In the ever-expanding digital landscape, safeguarding sensitive information and maintaining robust cybersecurity practices have become paramount. "Unveiling Cybersecurity Governance: Building a Strong Foundation" is a comprehensive guide that delves into cybersecurity governance's core principles and components, equipping readers with the knowledge and tools to establish a secure digital environment.

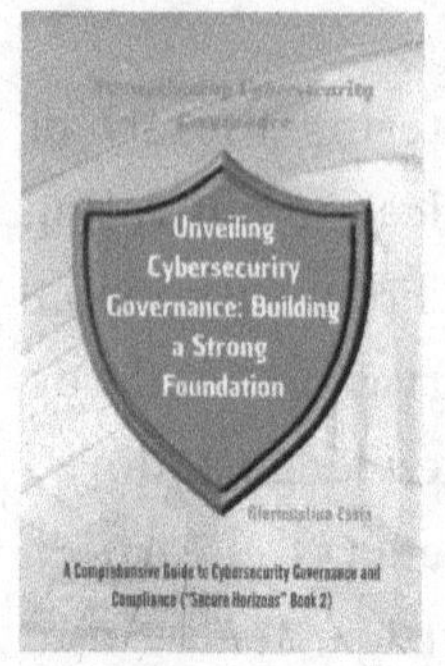

Unveiling Cybersecurity Governance

Step into a world where cybersecurity governance catalyzes a secure future. Explore the realms of "The Guardians of Security: Exploring the Role of Governance," the much-awaited second book in the epic series "Secure Horizons: A Comprehensive Guide to Cybersecurity Governance and Compliance."

As you read each page of "The Guardians of Security," prepare to be enchanted by the author's remarkable storytelling ability. This book presents a vivid picture of the complicated landscape of cybersecurity governance with a seamless blend of real-world experiences, cutting-edge research, and visionary concepts. Immerse yourself in an exciting story that uncovers the brains and souls of people dedicated to defending our digital borders.

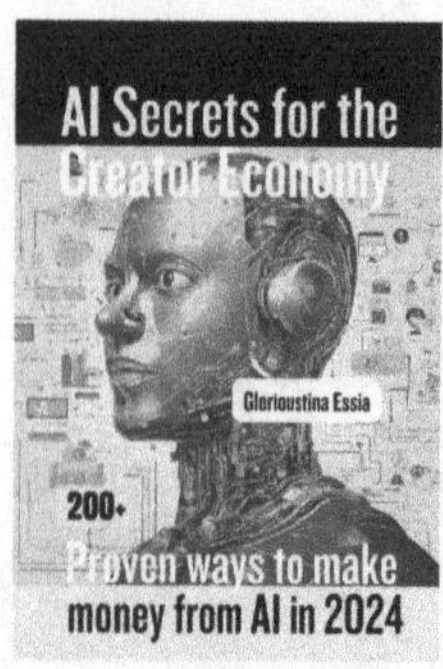

AI Secrets for the Creator Economy: 200+ Proven ways to make money from AI in 2024

In a world driven by innovation and transformation, the Creator Economy emerges as a powerful force, with Artificial Intelligence (AI) at its beating heart. This book, "AI Secrets for the Creator Economy: 200+ Proven Ways to Make Money from AI in 2024 and Beyond," is more than just a book; it's your key to unlocking the incredible synergy between AI and creativity, opening the door to a wealth of opportunities for those who are willing to seize them.